MW00461971

The Rhythms
of
Wellness

The Rhythms
of
Wellness

Follow the wisdom of the ancient sages and align with
Nature's cycles for greater health and wellbeing.

Jaki Daniels

Heartblight Publishing
CALGARY, ALBERTA

Hearthlight Publishing, Calgary, Alberta, Canada.

© 2018 Jaki Y. Daniels

First Softcover Edition December 2020
Library and Archives Canada Cataloguing in Publication Data

Daniels, Jaki Y. 1957–

The Rhythms of Wellness/ Jaki Daniels

ISBN: 978-0-9784636-6-3 (softcover)

EDITING AND PROOFREADING: Miranda Buchanan, Marilyn Geddes, Chris Daniels, Jay Daniels, Calgary, Alberta.

TYPESETTING & PRE-PRESS PRODUCTION: Chris Daniels

FINAL EDITING: Sandy Gough, Calgary, Alberta.

ILLUSTRATIONS: Nancy Kay, Redwood Meadows, Alberta

COVER DESIGN: Chris & Jaki Daniels

www.jakidaniels.com

Acknowledgements

Even when the book is small there are many hands who help to craft it. I'd like to express my deep appreciation to the following content editors who were a joy to work with: Chris Daniels, Jay Daniels, Miranda (Mica) Buchanan, and Marilyn Geddes. Also, thanks to Sandy Gough for her professional copy editing.

I'd like to thank Curtis Dillabough for being bold enough to suggest illustrations and, of course, to the artist Nancy Kay who drew them. She read, she contemplated, she dreamed, and brought the images to life.

When it came to developing the cover, Nancy Kay, Jay Daniels, and Mica Buchanan were enthusiastic and honest. Who could ask for more?

A special additional thank you to Mica Buchanan who in many ways held the vision of this book, and the value of its teachings, alive for me when I wasn't able to hold it for myself. She nudged and encouraged, reminded and cajoled, until it finally got completed.

In closing, a special acknowledgement must go to my husband Chris, who not only supports every project I embark upon, but is often the key person in the background making it happen. He was instrumental in every phase of this book's layout and publication.

Contents

	PREFACE	i
Chapter 1	INTRODUCTIONS	1
Chapter 2	MERIDIANS AND TIMING	9
	THE CHINESE CLOCK	12
Chapter 3	RECEIVING CHI FROM THE HEAVENS	15
Chapter 4	DRAINAGE AND DREGS	19
Chapter 5	ROTTING AND RIPENING	23
Chapter 6	DISTRIBUTION	29
Chapter 7	SUPREME CONTROLLER	33
Chapter 8	SEPARATING PURE FROM IMPURE	37
Chapter 9	CONTROL OF STORAGE	41
Chapter 10	CONTROL OF THE WATERWAYS	45
Chapter 11	HEART PROTECTOR	49
Chapter 12	THREE BURNING SPACES	53
Chapter 13	DECISION MAKING AND JUDGEMENTS	57
Chapter 14	PLANNING	59
Chapter 15	THE CHINESE CLOCK AS MEDICINE	63
Chapter 16	PLANNING FOR CHANGE	67
Chapter 17	ALIGNING TO THE CYCLES OF THE SUN	71
Chapter 18	MORE ON FOOD AND THE SEASONS	75
	AFTERWORD	81
	APPENDIX: HOW DO I BEGIN?	85

The Ancient Chinese Sages contributed their wisdom to the development of Classical Chinese Medicine, now in use for more than 4,000 years. This science is based on the elements that support our survival and the laws of nature. One key to wellness is in our understanding of these laws and our ability to follow them. Each step taken brings us closer to the vitality we all seek.

I have chosen to present this small book in the form of a conversation between the eager student and the Wise Sage, to replicate the teaching style of the Old Ways, when the apprentice was privileged to learn at the feet of the Master.

PREFACE

In 2013, when I first wrote the manuscript for this book, I had become intrigued with the Chinese Clock and created a project for myself of delving more deeply into understanding it. At that time there wasn't much talk about body rhythms in everyday conversation and I had no idea that was about to change. In 2017 the Nobel Prize in Physiology or Medicine was jointly awarded to Jeffrey C. Hall, Michael Rosbash, and Michael W. Young, for their discoveries of molecular mechanisms controlling the circadian rhythm. Over the space of the next few years modern society became increasingly aware of how intimately linked we are to the natural world around us and how body functions operate in coordinated patterns.

The award presentation posted on the Nobel Prize website states, "Their discoveries explain how plants, animals and humans adapt their biological rhythm so that it is synchronized with the Earth's revolutions" and, "With exquisite precision, our inner clock adapts our physiology to the dramatically different phases of the day. The clock regulates critical functions such as behavior, hormone levels, sleep, body temperature and metabolism. Our wellbeing is affected when there is a temporary mismatch between our external environment and this internal biological clock . . . There are also indications that chronic misalignment between our lifestyle and the rhythm dictated by our inner timekeeper is associated with increased risk for various diseases."

Since then all manner of media regularly discuss the topic, and words such as circadian and chronobiology are commonplace. I've seen articles with titles such as, "Eat more calories in the morning to lose weight", and heard experts say things like, "Our organs have their own clocks", or "The circadian rhythm has to be kept center and foremost." There is even evidence that the size of our brain shrinks while we sleep and that medications taken at different times of the day will have different effects in potency. We have quickly adjusted to what we believe is new science, yet the Chinese Sages were incorporating this knowledge into their system of medicine literally thousands of years ago.

What's more, in Classical Chinese Medicine, which focuses not only on organ systems but the meridians which support and provide life-force to those organs, it is recognized that the affects of this timing reach beyond the physical into how we think and how we feel on an emotional and spiritual level.

Today, in 2020, this little book is finally being published. My hope is that the focus on physiological timing over recent years will serve to ease you into these teachings and that you'll marvel that all this was known and mapped out so long ago. For me, our current scientific and medical knowledge only adds to the beauty and wisdom of the Chinese Clock.

Chapter 1

INTRODUCTIONS

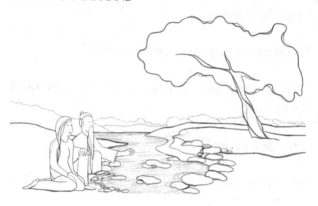

Imeet the Sage sitting by a creek, a small, clear, beautifully flowing creek with many pebbles on its banks. He is a slender man with a long white beard, gently pointed at the bottom and reaching down to his waist.

He speaks to me and says, "Welcome Little One. Come and sit."

At first I feel a little awkward. Do I perch among the small stones as he does? I hesitate, then realize I just need to follow his instructions so I sit down on the rocks, to his right. He wastes no time, immediately looking into my eyes. I sense that he is seeing into every part of me: physical, mental, emotional . . .

1

I had intended to formally introduce myself, which now seems unnecessary. Instead I ask simply, *"Great Sage, are you willing to teach me?"*

"Yes," he responds.

"What type of study are we to venture into?"

"A study of the life force that animates and enlivens all living beings."

"How do we begin?"

"We begin with the cycles of nature. Listen carefully:

In the night, much is still and quiet. The nocturnal creatures may be active but seldom are they loud. They go about their tasks allowing you to sleep. As the sun peeks its face over the horizon the world in its path becomes alive: activity and noise begin. The rooster crows at the crack of dawn. The children awake, hungry and thirsty, then ready to run and play. The cycles of the sun influence your internal cycles. If you follow these cycles, if you honour them, you will notice this supports your functioning in a very tangible way. You are familiar with taking medicines to soothe your ills; sometimes you even accompany those medicines with changes in patterns, habits and lifestyle. What if changing the patterns could *be* the medicine? What if

2

you could improve your health, well-being, and functionality in all ways—physical, emotional, mental, and spiritual—by adjusting your cycles and patterns to be supported by what is happening in the world outside?

"If you want to plant a garden, would you do it in winter? Would you move aside the blanket of snow, plant the seeds, cover them up and wait? What will happen if you plant your garden in the winter? Well, the seeds know what to do. They know how to grow into a plant. But they need the support of nature, they need the appropriate timing. If you plant your garden in the winter it will wait until spring to sprout and grow. If you plant your garden in the spring it will sprout and grow readily, and you will see the first shoots emerging from the earth in about ten days. If you use your garden to feed your family, when is the ideal time to plant if you are hoping for a speedy harvest?

"With this brief introduction can you begin to see how following the cycles and patterns, the timing of nature, can be of benefit?"

"Oh yes Sage, I most certainly can! Please continue."

"The cycles of light are powerful influences over living creatures and living forms, and are one of the most direct and immediate influences on your cycles. As part of nature, people have internal clocks, internal

3

mechanisms which are guided by the light, the sun. Just as creatures hibernate in winter and people sleep at night, the light of day holds within it a much ignored series of additional cycles that promote and support health and longevity. These teachings will serve to highlight those other cycles and guide you in using them to your healthful advantage.

"Some cycles of life are known to all. You move through the phases of infancy, childhood, adulthood, and elderhood. The cycles of the seasons take you through the year, from winter through spring to summer and fall. It is the angle of the changing light in the sky which creates a season—nothing more. The orbit of the earth around the sun, its distance from the sun at any given time, affects the earth and its inhabitants profoundly. In your day-to-day lives, the rising, setting, and angles of the sun have a similar influence. There are cycles and seasons which you go through each day and night.

"Humans function at their best when they are awake, alert, and active during the day and sleep soundly and sufficiently at night. When the sun first rises it is low on the horizon. At midday it is at its peak or arch. A daily sun cycle follows a similar path in the skies as it does during the seasons. There is a springtime in the morning: a fresh start, a new day. There is summer at noon: the fullest amount of light and activity you will have all day. At sunset there is autumn, winding down;

and at night there is winter: sleep, rest, and quiet in the darkness.

"There are seasons of the year, seasons of your lives, and seasons of your day.

"The life-force, growth, health, and vibrancy of the natural world are influenced by the sun. The same qualities within you, determined by your life-force, are influenced by the sun. The ancient Chinese followed the cycles of the seasons to learn about the changing patterns and the flow of nature. The sages and mystics explored both the physical and non-physical changes. They were able to see the blood on the physical level, its transportation network of veins, arteries, and capillaries. Those with the gift of inner sight were able to see the pathways of life-force that coursed through your bodies. They were also able to see the channels and network though which they travelled. They called these pathways, meridians.

"Ancient peoples around the earth were constantly studying their environment: the plants, the animals, the skies. Through knowing the cycles and their nuances they were able to understand their world. Their approach was one of relationship. What could be known, what could be understood, would help them to live well. Their focus was not limited to what they could see on the outside; they applied their attention and wisdom to what they could feel on the inside. Who you refer to as mystics, seers, or medicine people spent years developing their gifts of inner awareness. They meditated, contemplated, pondered, took themselves into trances and other varied states of spiritual experiences.

"Over many hundreds and thousands of years, through relationship with the visible and invisible world that affected all deeply and profoundly, patterns that supported survival and basic needs were noted. What was the best time of the day to hunt? What about gathering herbs? The ancient herbalists recognized that there are peak times for medicinal properties of plants, just as there are peak seasons for harvest. The Sages took this wisdom and applied it to human functions. What is the best time of day or night to make decisions? What is the best time of day to be active? In the same way that calendars were created from the cycles of the sun and the patterns of the sky, a calendar of internal function and energy flow was created. The Chinese called this pattern the Law of Midday/Midnight or the Chinese Clock.

"Have you ever heard someone say, "I need to sleep on it"? The ancient Chinese discovered that the function within you of decision making and judgement is related to the cycle of your life-force that is most active during the night, after you fall asleep. You may know from experience that you compromise your ability to make sound judgements and decisions if you do not sleep well. You also know that you don't function as well if you work during the night and sleep during the day.

"Some of the patterns they discerned have been remembered and practised through time. Some have been forgotten. But the wisdom has not been lost. It may have been buried in the excitement and possibilities of analytical science but your biology has not changed. The cycle of the seasons and the path of the sun across the sky is still the same as it was. You can choose to apply these principles in your life. You can allow nature's changing cycles and patterns to support your own functionality, specifically in terms of your health and well-being.

"In your next lessons we will look at the cycles and patterns of life-force flow throughout the day and night and learn what benefit will come to you through following them."

Chapter 2

MERIDIANS AND TIMING

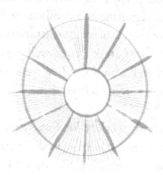

"*Sage, before we begin, can you offer instruction on the nature of the meridians in the body? How do they relate, in a practical way, to the cycles of nature of which we are a part?*"

"The key features of life are movement and energy. The storehouse for this capacity is understood in Chinese medicine to be the meridians and their associated vessels. The meridians are the pathways or channels of this life-force energy, which is sometimes referred to as Chi.

"The originators of this system of medicine were relational scientists who looked at the nature of life, the quality and quantity of life-force energy, and the relationship between that energy and functionality. Not just at the physical level—on all levels. You do not merely function as anatomical machines: you have thoughts, feelings, mood, character, personality, preferences, talents and creativity. These are as much a feature of life as digesting and eliminating. And people who are ill have less capacity for the variety of dynamic expressions in these areas than a well person. When you don't feel well you don't live well. When your vitality is compromised so is your joy.

"The intricate framework of life-force energy patterns reveals that each meridian has a peak functioning time and a low functioning time within a 24-hour cycle, the time it takes for one revolution of the earth. The inherent 'purpose' of each meridian flows through the body in phases and stages like the rising and falling of a wave. Each function within you comes into fullness like the crest, rising and contributing for two hours, then crashing as the momentum is passed along to the next meridian. When each meridian has made its contribution, the cycle begins again, to keep you functioning day after day.

"The Chinese Clock is the chart of these functions. "

THE CHINESE CLOCK

Peak Time	Meridian Function (and related organ)	Low Time
3:00am–5:00am	Receiving Chi from the Heavens (Lungs)	3:00pm–5:00pm
5:00am–7:00am	Drainage and Dregs (Colon)	5:00pm–7:00pm
7:00am–9:00am	Rotting and Ripening (Stomach)	7:00pm–9:00pm
9:00am–11:00am	Distribution (Spleen/Pancreas)	9:00pm–11:00pm
11:00am–1:00pm	Supreme Controller (Heart)	11:00pm–1:00am
1:00pm–3:00pm	Separating Pure from Impure (Small Intestine)	1:00am–3:00am

Peak Time	Meridian Function (and related organ)	Low Time
3:00pm–5:00pm	Control of Storage (Bladder)	3:00am–5:00am
5:00pm–7:00pm	Control of the Waterways (Kidneys)	5:00am–7:00am
7:00pm–9:00pm	Heart Protector (functional only)	7:00am–9:00am
9:00pm–11:00pm	Three Burning Spaces (functional only)	9:00am–11:00am
11:00pm–1:00am	Decision Making and Judgements (Gall Bladder)	11:00am–1:00pm
1:00am–3:00am	Planning (Liver)	1:00pm–3:00pm

Chapter 3

RECEIVING CHI FROM THE HEAVENS.

(Related Organ: Lungs)

Related Element: METAL

PEAK TIME: 3:00am–5:00am
LOW TIME: 3:00pm–5:00pm

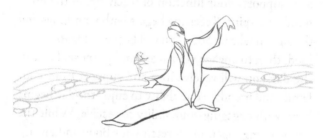

It is early dawn and I arrive at the creek in the forest before the sun is cresting the horizon. As I catch my first glimpse of the Sage today I notice he is doing movements with his arms, very beautiful, purposeful movements, similar to what I know as Qigong. A blue and white bird is playfully dodging and darting around his hands, as if anticipating each move then quickly getting out of the way. I call out to get his attention. *"Good morning Sage. I am here to begin my training in the Chinese Clock."*

"Good morning Little One! As you can see, it is the breaking of the dawn. Time to stretch and open the meridian flow for the day ahead. Before you take in your morning food you need to open yourself to the sun and engage your purpose and flow. This is the time of awakening, not just getting out of bed. Breathe! Enjoy the moment. Be grateful that the sun has risen to bring you warmth and light. Be grateful for your life. You have been given the gift of another day.

"This time is called Receiving Chi from the Heavens, as it supports your function of receiving, in the body, mind, and spirit. Receiving begins with your lungs and the air you take in. Soon you will be preparing to receive food, then to engage your work and purpose. Later in the day you will receive love and support from your family and friends. Your ability to enjoy the day begins here, with engaging your ability to receive. While the sun is rising, open up. Stretch your body and engage its physical strength and flexibility. Breathe deeply to enliven your blood. Extend and relax your limbs to open the meridians so they will know of this new beginning and can prepare for their peak time ahead.

"The inherent anticipation and excitement of a new day, of a new beginning, will carry you through. Let the earth and sky support and inspire you! Ride the wave of what is going on all around you—many inhabitants of the earth are waking up and preparing to receive the day.

"Perhaps if your days are dull, it is because you are not open to this kind of help. If you sleep late you will miss the opportunity this phase of the day provides. If you rise at 10:00am, no wonder you are not excited about the day. You missed your opportunity to be carried on nature's back. You didn't get inspired; you missed the peak time for cleansing and re-fuelling. At 10:00am your being is set to distribute nourishment but you haven't yet provided it with any.

"The lung time is a wondrous time of the day. Wake up. Breathe. Take it in. Feel yourself receive. Without this receiving from the sky you would weaken and expire within minutes. Yet if you fully engage your 'inspiration' in the morning, your day will hold much more for you than survival."

"Thank you Sage. Your teachings are wise and beautiful and I am privileged to receive them. Yet I also know that 'receiving' is just the beginning. I need to bring them forward into my day."

Chapter 4

DRAINAGE AND DREGS

(Related Organ: Colon)

Related Element: METAL

 PEAK TIME: 5:00am–7:00am
LOW TIME: 5:00pm–7:00pm

"*Sage, the next meridian on the Chinese Clock cycle is responsible for the function called Drainage and Dregs. Please explain.*"

"As the day breaks and the sun is close to the horizon, its light is cast upon the face of the earth. This building light is a signal to many creatures and life-forms to awaken and begin their day. This is naturally followed by movement and activity. We do not meet the day lying down! This movement and level of alertness sends signals to the body that help it prepare. It will need to eat and drink. It will need fuel for the day ahead. But first it must eliminate what is left behind. It must cleanse of the old to prepare for the new. The colon reveals this meridian's functionality through the efficiency and ease of the early morning bowel movement and elimination. Ah, now you can move into your day. Now you are ready to receive what the day brings. If you are clogged and full you cannot take in any more. Emptying prepares the way.

"At the level of the mind your thoughts look ahead to the day before you. In order to embrace the possibilities this day will bring you need to stop thinking about yesterday. Holding on to thoughts and feelings of the past will hold you back from receiving the fullness of today. Notice what the present moment is offering you.

"Also, there may have been times past when you were not able to fully express how you were feeling and it has stayed with you. Grief is one such emotion. If you do not express your grief fully in the days when it is all-consuming, you will not process and digest it, and the steps that need to be taken for efficient elimination will be stalled. If you hold on for too long, it will consti-pate you on levels other than the physical. Observing and being part of what is happening in the outside world can support this release. If you stop for a few minutes and watch the dawn, even from your window, you will feel the momentum to move forward, not stay behind. If you watch the sun peek over the horizon and spread light and warmth everywhere you will be affected by this. You will receive the subtle encourage-ment from nature to do the same. When your days are not supported by the changing skies they can all start to blur into one another. There will be no spark of shining light in the morning, no sunshine in your eyes. Over time your heart will become heavy from the absence of light-ness and change. Allow the light and the changing skies to inspire you and shift you. All you have to do is expose yourself instead of shielding against it. Watch the sunrise. Begin your day well."

Chapter 5

ROTTING AND RIPENING
(Related Organ: Stomach)

Related Element: EARTH

 PEAK TIME: 7:00am–9:00am
LOW TIME: 7:00pm–9:00pm

A s I arrive at the creek the blue and white bird flies over to where the Chinese Sage is standing and hovers near him for a while. The Sage sits down, facing me. "It is a joy to share these details with you. There are not many who are interested enough to ask!"

"Thank you Sage. I treasure this natural wisdom and the traditional teachings that have been neglected or forgotten. Today may we focus on the function of Rotting and Ripening?"

"Oh Little One, the stomach time is a very important time of the day. There is much to learn. The stomach meridian is dedicated to taking in and digesting. This function is in response to need, as are all functions. For the system to have fuel and to operate at peak efficiency during the day it must have a 'fill-up' in the morning.

There needs to be a clean body, emptied of its waste to create the appetite and space to be filled.

"So first we look to the appetite. Many say they are not hungry in the morning. Then I say they should look to how closely they are following the cycles and the clock. For you to enjoy your food and enjoy your day you should have an appetite for it, be keen and ready for your fill-up. The appetite prepares the body, mind, and spirit. On the physical level the digestive juices are primed and ready to support. On the mental level you may be breaking up the tasks for the day into manageable chunks. On the spiritual level you are excited about the possibilities for wonder, growth, amusement and joy. The system is ready.

"The type of fuel needed for the physical level is food. The better the quality of food the more efficiently the system will function. Complexity and wholeness of foods are important here. Foods in their natural state that have not been processed, stripped of parts or refined, will provide the body with the challenge of digestion. A healthy meridian is like an elite athlete. It wants to work, it wants to perform and function in all the ways it has been designed for. Offering processed food denies the body's ability to break down complex food components and over time it will weaken from lack of use. The nature of the food itself is best determined by your planned activities for the day.

"If you are someone who works outside doing physical labour, your breakfast should be protein based, including some green leaves for minerals and some complex starch for energy. You need an efficient stomach to digest these in combination, but an efficient stomach will work diligently and carefully to manage your fuel supply well. For those who are scholars or thinkers, planners or leaders, whose minds are active while their bodies are still, a light quality protein will serve, such as a few ounces of fish with some vegetables or fresh greens. Artists, ask yourselves, are you feeding your physical bodies or your minds? Depending on the answer, your needs will be different. Creativity requires the support of live foods; again the body builds upon what nature is already providing to make the task easier. Fresh fruit and greens with sprouted seeds will provide the intense bursts of light and life that will be needed. And if you are a monk or a dedicated spiritual servant, be sure to bless your food and receive it in a prayer-full manner. If your daily tasks are to give to others of your own spirit, then begin your day by taking in an abundance of the Great Spirit—the One Spirit.

"Next, do not taint this valuable food, which is still whole, with stimulants that will alter the food's quality. Beware of any additive used in concentrated form. Salt and sugar are key agents here, another would be ground spices. These should be used sparingly, to brighten and increase appetite but not to distort the flavour of the food.

"Eat slowly and chew well, so that your body is aware on all sensory levels of the taste, texture, colour, flavour, and smell of the food. Appetite isn't just about filling the stomach; it is about engaging the senses and your awareness so that you may feel and experience the richness life offers. Think of it. Each food has a different texture, a different taste and smell. Does that not contribute to your enjoyment of life? Ignoring or bypassing the sensory appeal and satisfaction of food will lead to dullness within you, at all levels. Ah, the bite into a crisp apple and the release of its juices; the sweetness of a grain or root vegetable—the texture dense and hearty; the minerals of leaves and green foods; the tang of herbs; the satisfying chew of meat. Food is fuel and sensory delight. The honing and sharpening of your senses in your daily meals will heighten those senses at other times and for other uses.

"Food for the mind should be considered accordingly. What study or learning are you taking in? Is that study something that enriches your being? Be cautious here too. When the eyes/brain/mind have to process an excess of stimulation in a short period of time it will compromise and distort other functions in the same way that concentrated additives like salt and sugar can on the physical level. Any excess needs to be balanced or adjusted with rest and recovery. Those thinkers and planners who are expected to remain sharp and focus all day will need to pace their exertion and take care.

"And a day without food for the soul will limit your zest for life, your joy and enthusiasm. Take the time to watch the sunrise, marvel at the beauty of the season on your way to work, allow the awe and wonder of child-like innocence to fill you with feelings that reveal your deeper nature and character. What do you love? Who do you love? What does love feel like? Don't brush it away; don't take for granted that you can pay attention to it another time. Relish it now!"

Chapter 6

DISTRIBUTION
(Related Organs: Spleen/Pancreas)

Related Element: EARTH

 PEAK TIME: 9:00am–11:00am
LOW TIME: 9:00pm–11:00pm

"*G*reat Sage, will you speak about the function of *Distribution?*"

"What your stomach has received and prepared must now be distributed. What you have taken in and digested must now become available for your use, whether that food was for the mind, body, or spirit. Leaving it in the stomach serves no purpose. Everything you put into your body and everything your body creates from it, has to be moved to where it will do the most good. Within you is a network of channels so that transportation, distribution and flow are all possible. You are a living system of cycles. Food, blood, and all manner of body chemistry must travel to where they are needed. The function of distribution is the master of flow. This requires support, of course. There must be a plan, there needs to be appropriate timing, but we can discuss the others later. For now, we are focusing on where things need to go and the route they must take to get there.

"One can easily surmise how important this is; when you travel you need to know where you are going and how to get there. If you have been out gathering foods you need to get them home and into the cupboards, so you will have access when you need them. Certainly you have felt the frustration of needing something, being certain that the supply is at hand, and not being able to find it? Moment to moment this meridian is working to make the most of what you have available.

"This is also critical on a mental level. Without this function there will be times when it appears there's never enough information, never enough thinking it through, never the sense of taking a situation from conception to resolution. A person in whom this function is compromised will be prone to worry, staying on the wheel of churning the same thoughts, ideas, and conversations, around and around. They don't get taken to where they will best serve—the next level of understanding and comprehension.

"And in the heart? How do you make the most of what you have in life and feel content and satisfied? How do you work with what's available and feel that your needs are being met? Where is the 'assurance' quality in your functioning? Are you able to trust that what you have and what you are being given will meet your needs to a satisfactory level?

"Can you imagine the state of un-ease in the body when this distribution is compromised? What if your hormones, or other components of blood, are produced but don't get to where they are needed? Even the tools of science cannot look into the body and find all the chemistry that has been lost, stuck, taken to the wrong place or excreted as garbage when it hadn't been used yet! "Oops, I gave that away and now realize I need it!" Has this ever happened? Or perhaps you never gave any-thing away; instead you hoarded everything, and then can't easily find the one thing that you need because there is too much clutter to make it accessible. Effective distribution is critical."

Chapter 7

SUPREME CONTROLLER
(Related Organ: Heart)

Related Element: FIRE

 PEAK TIME: 11:00am–1:00pm
LOW TIME: 11:00pm–1:00am

I arrive in the forest. I look across the creek and see the Chinese Sage waiting for me and ready to begin. I call out a heartfelt *"Good Morning."*

"Sage, may we continue with the Chinese Clock? If we are following the path of the sun, our next meridian peak time is the Supreme Controller."

"The heart meridian is of the Fire Element so it is most appropriate that its peak time is when the sun is high in the sky. The sun is our daily reminder of the Fire Element and its light and warmth. The heart meridian is considered the Supreme Controller: the wise leader who rules the kingdom and maintains order. The ultimate expression of the Fire Element is Love. The heart and heart meridian allow an individual to experience love, to feel the fire within, and to be able to offer love and warmth to others because it is known and felt within one's self.

"To best support its efforts on your behalf you can assist by being outside during this phase of the day. How convenient that even people who work indoors can often go outside at midday for a walk or to eat. When the sun is at its peak of brightness so should you be. This is the ideal time for activity and exercise. The ancient Chinese considered that the pores of the body open to their fullest when the sun is highest in the sky, allowing your body to sweat, release any excess heat, and maintain balance. You should warm your bodies. You should encourage the pores to open and release any toxins which may be building up inside. A build-up of toxins can inhibit the flow of all meridians and therefore limit their expression and your function. Take some time to be outside. Feel the warmth of the sun cleansing your pores and your body, allowing for flow. This will help you to feel vital and that in turn will be noticed and received by others. So the Fire Element supports you, supports your relationships, and supports your heart on all levels: body, mind, and spirit.

"Of course, too much can be harmful, and the heat of day in the peak of summer can produce more heat in the body than you are able to adjust to and accommodate. It can parch, it can scorch, and it can burn.

When two peak expressions of nature come together it makes sense that the combination will be potent, and care needs to be taken. Be cautious. Be careful. Feel what it is that you need. Notice when it is too much.

"The meridian clock is an expression of light and flow. It is based on the timing of the sun. That is why the heart meridian is called the Supreme Controller. The light inherent in fire and the flow of warmth it encourages establish the flow for all the other meridians. The sun controls life outside. The Fire Element controls the life-force within you. When the sun has risen and is expressing itself fully, this signals and supports you in expressing yourself fully. This is when you should be active, dynamic, and productive.

"When the sun is rising or setting, or in the dark of night, it is time for quiet and rest. It is the clock of the sun that you should pay attention to. Activity in the day, peace and contemplation at night. The early morning and after dinner hours are not the ideal time for physical activity, particularly if it is strenuous. People who begin their activities and chores in the early morning before the sun is up are following an artificial cycle and not a natural one. Depending on the health and vitality of the other meridians, this could indeed compromise their overall function in some way. The effects cannot be generalized; each individual's expression of dis-ease will be unique to them because the expression of twelve meridians in a particular living system is complex and can contain infinite variations. Instead of trying to catalogue risks, let me instead encourage you to support your Supreme Controller in all the ways that you are able. It is wonderful to have your meridians held under the wise counsel of a Supreme Controller who rules with love, warmth, effective communication, consideration, and the intelligent understanding that when each meridian is empowered to do its job well and is provided with the life-force energy to do just that, the system can function at its peak of power and performance. A system operates best as a system, not as independent parts that are not aware of the possibilities of the functional 'whole'. If you want to be at your best, do all you can to support your Supreme Controller and it will do all it can to support you."

Chapter 8

SEPARATING PURE FROM IMPURE
(Related Organ: Small Intestine)

Related Element: FIRE

PEAK TIME: 1:00pm–3:00pm
LOW TIME: 1:00am–3:00am

"*S*age, *our next meridian is in charge of Sorting and Separating.*"

"The Small Intestine time is also Fire time. We are still in the heat of the day, so to speak. Fire provides energy, and the role of the small intestine meridian is to sort and separate: to provide for the body that which is supportive and nourishing, and release what is toxic. You will note that there are several mechanisms to receive and release in the body—remember the lungs and colon? They form the pair of the element Metal. It is important to differentiate the role of the small intestine meridian, however, as the 'sort' function is key. Decisions must be made as to what to keep and what to let go of. These decisions are based on value. The body strives to be an efficient system with no excess and with regular garbage disposal. It determines the value of what is to be kept, what is to be used as fuel and nourishment, and what are to be the building blocks for the growth of your mind, body, and spirit. This requires the element of Fire so that love, warmth, and wise management serve as the foundation for these decisions.

"It is no accident that the small intestine time follows the Supreme Controller time. The system requires competent rule and an efficiently functioning team. The peak time of the Supreme Controller leads into the finer nature of deciding the raw materials the kingdom requires to carry out the multitude of tasks. If there is filth in the system it can get clogged. In an already dirty system, more dirt goes unnoticed, so the conditions for addiction to unhealthy substances can flourish. When the system is pure and clean, and value is sought out and received so gratefully that every morsel is utilized, then dirt becomes offensive.

"The pure and clean body, mind, and spirit are not attracted to dirt and perversion. Do you see? Once dirt has settled in, found a place, more dirt does not signal the alarm. A person who has never smoked and inhales their first cigarette will become ill. A person who smokes heavily will barely notice the effect of smoking more. This goes for many areas of influence. We could begin with food; we could look at violence, pornography, abuse, hatred and prejudice against others. The role of the small intestine meridian is to sort the pure from the impure, the nourishing from the toxic and harmful. Purity in itself is an extreme, but you have a built-in margin of allowance which keeps you within a range of normal healthy functioning. Some impurities are expected and handled easily.

"In the small intestine meridian, the pure essence of love is distilled down into the selection of that which best supports a Being of Love, and that role, that function, is to hang on to what nourishes and to let go of that which can build up, clog, and pollute."

Chapter 9

CONTROL OF STORAGE
(Related Organ: Bladder)

Related Element: WATER

 PEAK TIME: 3:00pm–5:00pm
LOW TIME: 3:00am–5:00am

" *A nd what about from 3:00–5:00pm, when our Storage function reaches its peak?*"

"The bladder meridian is all about storage. You store what you need until it is time to be released. Again we see that this function carries over into organs not directly associated with the bladder meridian. In a sense the colon stores also and releases when the time is right. We can observe from the function of these two systems where there is dysfunction in your society. Diarrhea, constipation, and weak bladder are rampant. Whereas once only adversely affected during illness or infections, these are now daily occurrences among you. Many people are not storing and releasing wisely. They hold on for too little or too long. When they do

41

eliminate, it is often incomplete, not resulting in the satisfaction a full emptying can provide.

"Once you have determined what to hold onto through the sort and separating function, you need a method of storage. The bladder time could not arrive at a better moment. The ability to store wisely, to have 'stores' managed efficiently so there is always enough in times of need, these are managed through this meridian. If you take in more than you need, the size of the body will have to increase. If you store it for too long, it will no longer be at its prime; it will start to degrade. If the storage facilities are not clean and of themselves functioning well, they can contribute to contamination. So again, storage is not limited to one organ. But the function of storage, the mastermind behind storage, is the bladder meridian. You are not always consciously aware, at any given point in time, if the colon is storing well. But you are acutely aware of the bladder. Its signals cannot be ignored. 'Time to empty' and 'room for more' are easily and continually noticed. On an expanded level, it's also an indicator of how much you want to take into your life. Look around your culture—bigger homes, bigger closets, bigger pantries. How much do you really want to store? And what about storage facilities that allow people to store more than they can possibly hold within their own living space? What does this say? What about taking only what you need and leaving the rest for others? Here we can see into the wisdom of the bladder meridian. It not only functions as storage; it determines what and how much needs to be stored. Such a valuable function.

"This brings us to another feature of the Water Element. The emotions we spoke of related to Fire were love and warmth. The emotion related to Water is fear. The more fearful you are the more you will want to store—just in case! This underlying fear leads to all kinds of storage problems. It is well known that a sign of acute fear is uncontrolled urination. There are also others who dribble, never quite holding on. A little comes in—a little goes out. How can you boldly step forward if you are not assured of your reserves? But ah, we are moving onto the next phase of our cycle, the kidneys . . ."

Chapter 10

CONTROL OF THE WATERWAYS
(Related Organ: Kidneys)

Related Element: WATER

 PEAK TIME: 5:00pm–7:00pm
LOW TIME: 5:00am–7:00am

"The meridian in control of your waterways is also the holder of your ancestral Chi. It is the guardian of the lineage that begot you. Each person's life begins from the essence of two others, mother and father, and the quality, quantity, and purity of that essence is their gift to you. After conception, the mother can help you grow and be nourished in your fetal development but your ancestral essence has already been established and remains unchanged. This is your inheritance. Any good parent would hope to see you spend it wisely and for it to contribute value in your life. Your inheritance cannot be increased once received. Your parents gave you all they had to give. Your inheritance cannot be shared. It provided the foundation of your life-force, and only yours. But it can be squandered. You can spend it recklessly, taking it for granted and expecting that it will never truly run out.

"There is also the fund of life-force energy which you contribute to. The quality of your air, breath, food, and fuel all have the possibility to contribute essence, in quantity and quality, and it is these stores that are your fuel on a daily basis. The ancestral inheritance is your savings, your reserves. The Chinese studied for thousands of years to develop an understanding of how best to maintain this inheritance. They developed methods of movement that kept the body and life-force flowing but did not exhaust or deplete. They considered their own sexual fluids as part of their inheritance, being of their own essence, and chose to keep their sexual activities to a considered and reasonable amount. All the ways they kept a close watch on their inheritance are the same ways your people have available to them now. This has not changed over time. How carefully do you manage your inheritance, your essence, your life force? Do you take care that your daily air and food provide for your expenditures so you do not dip into the reserves? Or do you eat to excess, drink alcohol to excess, partake of poor quality food and drink, stay up late, and otherwise neglect your true needs?

"In your bodies water is life, and therefore your supplies of water, the quality of water, and the proper mainten-ance of water and all fluids is critical. You can see how the function of the kidney meridian, which controls the waterways, would be so closely related to your inherited life force. Maintaining fluids and guarding your Chi are both critical to your life and your level of function.

"So far, the day has been about building and fuel. It has been about growth and expression. You rose, you ate, you were active while the sun was high, and now, as the sun starts to decline, it is time to ensure that all you have gathered is held in the wise control of this meridian. Now the management of your funds can begin in earnest. As your day's activities draw to a close, you too can review and consider what your efforts and your work have provided and how to manage it well. If you continue your activity and work into the later part of the day and evening, management becomes more difficult. The person who does this will start to lose sight of how much they actually need, and, in an effort to have enough, will just keep earning and accumulating more. Alternately, a person who does not bring themselves forward, who does not contribute or serve during the day, will constantly be turning to others for help and support, because their needs are greater than what they are able to provide for themselves.

"It is not meant for you to hoard your ancestral Chi. It is there to contribute quality and quantity to your life-force energy. It is there to support you in functioning in all the ways you are able, which includes work, gathering fuel, elimination, storage, management, distribution, joy, laughter, sharing and bonding with others, effective communication, intimacy, passion, wise counsel, and more. To live a full and balanced life these qualities must all have a place."

Chapter 11

HEART PROTECTOR
(Related organ: None)

Related Element: FIRE

 PEAK TIME: 7:00pm–9:00pm
LOW TIME: 7:00am–9:00am

"*S*age, may we move into Heart Protector time?"

"At the end of the water time we move into heart nourishing time. These next two cycles are critical for the sound functioning of the emotional and spiritual heart, as well as the distribution of blood and heat. You have nourished your body and taken care of its needs. You have been awake and alert; you have been active and in service. Now you must take care of yourself and your loved ones and they in turn, can enrich you. We move into family time and gathering together as the sun is in its descent. It is time for the heart to be filled with love and to express joy, attraction, creativity, and sharing. It is time to play with the children after a day of work, to light the fire and share the stories. It is time to laugh and feel loved.

"If you do not appreciate and embrace this time you will surely be harming yourselves. One of the riches of sharing love is that it warms you on the inside and provides for the efficient flow of blood. As you enter into the states of joy and ease, your blood and life-force meet, supporting the blood's ability to circulate. This circulation and warmth, combined with the emotional bonding, opens the way for intimacy and the pleasures of deep, soul-full attraction. This is also the time of day that is easily given up. The worker in the family stays late and does not share in this time with their partner and children. This is also a time of transportation and separation of family members as children are taken to their evening activities. Do you see how this compromises several features of the cycle? Activities are left until late in the day when the pores are starting to close. Family time becomes fragmented; the settling into play and leisure together is sacrificed for the desire to fill your lives with so much variety and purpose. This is not seen as unusual. Yet truly you simply need to be who you are; to be vital, to eat well, to rest well, and to share the joys of heart and community.

"This is also a time when the natural, inherent gifts of the children come to light. As families spend time together and play together, they see into each other's character and true nature. The aptitudes of the children are revealed, and once known, they can be nurtured by the family and greater community. When activities are planned ahead and scheduled by the mind they can sometimes override the subtle, natural gifts that are waiting for encouragement and support. Sadly, this is also a time when parents can be exhausted, and children can be an additional challenge at the end of a day that has already been depleting.

"Each part of the cycle feeds into the next: if you don't sleep well; if you don't rise and clean yourself of waste; if you don't eat, move your body, then contribute your talents and gifts in a productive way, you will not feel the pleasure and joy that sharing provides at the day's close. You will not be ready to share of yourself as there are other needs to be met. This in turn compromises your blood flow, the viscosity of your bodily fluids, and the warmth you feel in your heart."

Chapter 12

THREE BURNING SPACES
(Related Organ: None)

Related Element: FIRE

 PEAK TIME: 9:00pm–11:00pm
LOW TIMES: 9:00am–11:00am

"We then move into Triple Warmer time, another form of distribution. The warmth that is being generated must be made available to all parts of the body so that you function at your best and at the ideal internal temperature. As with all life-force function, this benefit is not limited to the physical. This meridian also ensures that you function at the ideal emotional temperature, that the warmth you feel in your heart is abundant and there is no need to hold back in sharing it with others. When some appear cold and heartless, it is often because the cycle has been violated and you haven't been provided with your basic needs so the warmth will flourish. Love and affection are meant to be shared. It is inherent in their nature.

"The Triple Warmer function allows for the three divisions of the body to receive an equal amount of warmth and maintain a consistent optimal temperature, despite external influences. This is a very important task. If the upper body is hot and the lower body is hotter or colder, function will be compromised. The Triple Warmer also distributes warmth to the three layers of your being: body, mind, and spirit. It is important that your level of warmth be as consistent throughout these layers as it is in the physical divisions. The mind needs to make decisions based on care and compassion for others. Cold hard decisions may serve a financial or economic bottom line but seldom a humane one. In fact, it is often the intention of cold, hard decisions to bypass any sensitive or emotional considerations.

"There are times when the external conditions are extreme, and the body cannot maintain even heating throughout, as in the case of frostbite. The tissue can no longer sustain its warmth and succumbs to the cold. There are diseases of circulation where the tissue in the limbs becomes infected and rotting. The life-force energy cannot be sustained there. There are emotional conditions where the uneven distribution of warmth becomes evident; there is heightened and intense sexuality or sexual activity with no warmth in the heart. An opposite condition can also manifest: plenty of affection from the heart and the mind but no desire for sexual intimacy. Sometimes the heart is warm and the womb is cold, leading to infertility. There are multitudes of ways that uneven distribution of warmth can compromise. Life functions best with a precise, even temperature throughout. Your Triple Warmer function serves this purpose and operates at its peak between 9:00pm and 11:00pm. The sun has set and all its fire, warmth and passion are safely absorbed and tucked inside, shared equally with all the different sections and layers, and you are comfortable, warm, joyful, and loving—a blissful state to take into your dream time."

Chapter 13

DECISION MAKING AND JUDGEMENTS
(Related Organ: Gall Bladder)

Related Element: WOOD

PEAK TIME: 11:00pm–1:00am
LOW TIME: 11:00am–1:00pm

"As we move into the time of decision making and judgements it is only fitting that we take into our decisions all the fuel, warmth, and love that the day has brought us. From that place of contentment and restful sleep, the Fire Element has laid the foundation for wise and clear counsel. The day has seen your active, physical manifestations; the night sees the more internal ones.

"There are functions within you that allow for articulate and well-conceived decisions to be made, to serve the organism in its many duties and activities in the days ahead. There needs to be physical rest in the body for these inner functions to operate at their peak. The internal 'boardroom' where these decisions are made must be calm and quiet to operate efficiently and effectively. If the body is restless, or the mind or spirit, it will be disruptive to this meridian's function. Those who stay up late or do not sleep peacefully will have difficulty with their decisions, both the timeliness of them and their quality. These decisions are not just mental ones; there are moment-to-moment decisions that are molecular and physical that must be carried out to keep the body functioning well.

"Remember there is sorting and separating to do; there is distribution of nutrients, cells, blood, and hormones; there is effective rule and leadership; there is circulation and warmth. All functions of the cycle support each other and decisions need to be made for all of them. You must function well in your decision making to be vibrant, happy, healthy, and functional in all the ways possible. The internal boardroom must be clear and uncluttered, calm not chaotic, organized and spacious, to allow creativity room to flow. This can be one of the easiest phases of the cycle to honour. You simply need to be asleep before 11:00pm. When you wake up in the morning you will begin making decisions from the moment you open your eyes, so you need this time to prepare."

Chapter 14

PLANNING
(Related Organ: Liver)

Related Element: WOOD

 PEAK TIME: 1:00am–3:00am
LOW TIME: 1:00pm–3:00pm

"The next phase of the cycle is the peak time for the function of planning. The liver meridian is the master planner and nothing works well without a plan in place. However, the planner needs to be able to trust the team, to have some assurance that the plan can be received without distortion. This is why the planning time follows the decision making time. When the planner is assured that decisions can be carried out wisely and effectively, with flexibility in times of surprise or unpredictability, then the plans can be handed over with trust and confidence.

"Confidence is a key feature of the liver meridian and the function of planning. No one wants to begin developing a plan without the confidence it will be carried out. The plan provides a strong foundation and allows for appropriate timing and balance. When there is no plan in place, at minimum you experience disruption, and in incremental degrees you move toward chaos. A wise and effective plan calms the mind and spirit. It enables ease and flow.

"The timing of your day and the timing of your cycles (both internal and external) need the function of this meridian. How well are you supporting it? Are you sleeping at the appropriate time? Are you unwinding and letting go in the evening: finishing your work and releasing your desire for food? A disruption anywhere in the cycle can begin here with the Wood Element, as it lays the foundation for appropriate quality and quantity of Chi flow.

"When decisions can be carefully and meticulously attended to, and the plan developed with clarity and purpose, you will be able to see ahead. You will be able to look into the future and sense what it will reap for you. Remember the garden and the timing of when to plant? Your mind can operate disconnected from nature's plan and you can plant your garden in the winter, but it will wait until the spring, the season of the Wood Element, for the plan inherent in each seed to become activated. Once you see the green shoots sprouting forth you can begin to look ahead to the resulting fruits, vegetables and flowers. You tend them carefully because if you are attentive to their needs, their simple elemental needs, you will receive a bounty to harvest. And so it is with your life. You will reap the rewards of what you have sown.

"If this phase of the clock is compromised can you see how frustration will result? All the decisions your body, mind and spirit require, for ease of functioning, all the best laid plans. . . If you do not support these functions, not only will your days appear disruptive, to yourself and others, your internal functioning will also. The emotion associated with the Wood Element is anger. Anger is borne of frustration. Frustration arises when things don't go according to plan, or when there is no well laid plan.

"The cycle requires your attention and respect. A plan requires your attention and respect. If you choose to ignore a plan or reject a plan, you will find yourself at the mercy of the other forces in your life. You will feel lost at times, lost and hopeless. The plan plants the seeds of hope.

"The entire clock runs smoothly when the plan is well conceived and the conditions allowed for its implementation are set. That is why this meridian functions at its best before the break of day. The plan has been laid, the timing has been established, the efforts to support the foundation of all your meridians are in place. When you wake up, you can begin your day well."

Chapter 15

THE CHINESE CLOCK AS MEDICINE

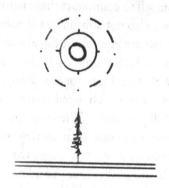

"*Sage, you have been so considerate in your teachings of the Chinese Clock. Can you help me to understand its use as medicine?*"

"Humans are complex beings. They have free will and can choose their actions and thoughts. They can go with the flow or go against it. They can live their lives in a way that acknowledges and nurtures that flow or they can make choices which hinder it.

"I am here to teach you about the naturally occurring cycles so you can use your free will wisely. In the time of your ancestors this was the only way to live that made sense—that was reasonable and rational. Now it requires thought and effort to align with the cycles. So I offer these teachings to support you. Implementing them is indeed a form of medicine.

"To allow yourself to counteract these natural cycles is to hinder flow. This not only limits the natural range of expressions that are possible, it can also contribute to opposing flow, which ultimately leads to a discordant pattern. Flow that has been stopped, plugged, interfered with, or at its worst—changed course, will directly affect *your* ability to flow. When you are not flowing, you will know it because your system will alert you. There is a built-in protective alarm that signals you to resume the natural course. You know this alarm system as symptoms. Your body, mind, and spirit will react when flow has been affected so you don't need to worry—as long as you pay attention!

"When those alarm signals are mild and in their early stages it is a simple matter to assess where flow has been interrupted. Resume course and you will be on your way, flowing smoothly again. If you ignore the alarm, over time the interrupted flow will begin to limit the internal mechanisms of function and healing.

"At its most initial stages, no 'doctor' is needed. Realign yourself with the powerful natural cycles of which you are a part and flow will be resumed. These are the teachings offered here. If your dis-ease has progressed beyond that point, or it is not possible for you to realign, then a practitioner of meridian balancing can offer adjustments and support. It is best that this practitioner serves to re-establish flow in its fullness and entirety and does not simply turn off the alarm. If the dis-ease has progressed beyond what a meridian specialist can correct, then your illness has progressed beyond what your life-force can naturally remedy. There are additional measures you can turn to, and at times this level of intervention can remove the obstacles that have built up to prevent flow and you will be given a second chance.

"There are also accidents and injuries with such impact that they are immediate obstacles to flow; they do not build up over time through the choices you have made. In some of these cases meridian realignment and correction can support your healing needs. Many times, however, more dramatic interventions may be indicated. Any intervention that removes obstacles to flow is potentially life-saving.

"The wise way to approach the re-establishment of your life-force flow and its expressions is to begin your corrections at the first sign of imbalance and choose the safest and most non-invasive method. There is no risk, no fee, and no adverse outcome to realigning yourself with the flow of nature. This, whenever possible, should be your first choice. If you pay attention to the alarm signals and realign when you have veered off course, you will be tapping into a system of supportive healing that is as powerful as nature herself."

Chapter 16

PLANNING FOR CHANGE

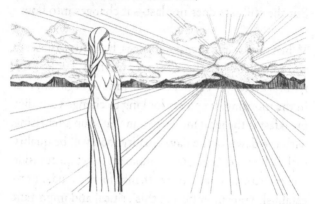

"*Sage, for many people, change is difficult. Sometimes change is scary. How do we find within ourselves what we need to make the necessary changes?*"

"Changes occur naturally. They are part of the flow of life. Nothing stays the same. One season flows into the next; the sun does not stay in one place—it moves across the sky. The clouds and weather patterns are not fixed; they are constantly moving and changing. Change is inherent in cycles and flow.

"But flow is not necessarily inherent in change—not in man. Man decides with the mind, goes against the natural cycles of flow and attempts to initiate change in a contrary manner. Then he is surprised that the changes do not flow—that there is resistance. The water in the river flows. The rate of flow may speed up or slow down. The water may even appear still at times. But the stillness does not last—it changes into flow.

"When man wants to make changes, he needs to observe and consider when these changes will flow. Look to the natural cycles for your cues! The time to begin anew is in the morning. If you are looking to change your diet, breakfast is the ideal meal to begin. Eat soon after rising, with the dawn of the day. Quality food will be quality fuel. Before you begin, take a moment to get quiet inside and prepare, not only to give thanks for the food, but to establish your intention at this critical and important time. The entry into the new day and the entry into the new way can align and support each other. A time of gratitude, meditation, or prayer brings your internal desires forward, places them into the world, and allows the intentions to become real.

"The next consideration is how to hold on to the change. As you move through your day, your body repeats its postures and patterns of the previous day. Your work and your tasks repeat the patterns also. This re-engagement can remind of the former state and create resistance to change. Therefore, the intention you placed upon yourself in the morning declaration must be supported throughout the day. You must provide an opening to allow it to grow and flourish. If the intention for change is only acknowledged for fifteen minutes in the morning, all can be undone by evening.

"The keys are posture and patterns, posture and patterns. If you change your daily posture and patterns you continue to create change, thereby establishing flow.

"During your morning time of opening and receiving, stand facing the sun. Ask for guidance on how the posture of your body can support your desired change. Feel what happens. Hold your intention in your heart and feel the way your body responds. Note this. Then with your inner sight look forward into your day—see the patterns you follow. Which ones will inhibit your change? If you cannot identify any patterns then perhaps there are none to release, but the need for change still exists. Decide on something different. Ten minutes outside during lunch, some stretches on your break, a cup of tea sipped in meditation. The 'new' isn't only a moment in time. Allow it to be a catalyst for continued change.

"Then identify the time of day that is most difficult for you. Is it late afternoon or evening? Your energy is waning, the sun is not as brilliant, all is winding down. The creativity moves from active to passive. What relaxing activity can you do that is outside your previous pattern? Can you sing, play music, draw? Can you do beadwork, darn socks, knit a sweater? Traditionally the end of the day is for relaxing, social, and art-full activities. A ten-minute drawing project can change the entire course of your evening and help break up the old patterns. Allow yourself those ten minutes. Surely there is something you have always wanted to do but didn't have the time. Begin there.

"As you retire for the evening, spend a few minutes in contemplation, meditation, or prayer—whatever suits you. Perhaps light a candle and sit quietly. Feel in your heart the changes you want to make and take the time to review all the positive contributions you have already made. Allow yourself to feel gratitude for those accomplishments. Do not engage in judgements and negativity. Do not bring these into your thoughts. There is always another day to try, so any entertainment of failure is too premature to take seriously. In the morning when the sun rises, you can begin again."

Chapter 17

ALIGNING TO THE CYCLES OF THE SUN

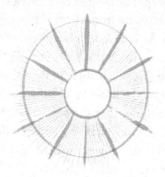

"*Sage, where I live the light of the sun changes slightly each day and dramatically through the seasons. How are we to follow the sun cycle as our clock when it changes so?*"

"I'm so pleased that you asked. The very question however, shows how far people have removed themselves from nature's cycles. The answer is so simple.

"You rise with the sun and sleep with the night. In between those times the features of your day will be the same. You rise with the dawn, take time to breathe, open your body and begin taking in Chi from the heavens. You will be preparing for your day will you not? Cleansing, eliminating, eating breakfast and then engaging your daily work. There will be maximum light in the middle of the day and you can be active. "There will also be an end to your work day and time to spend with friends and family. Then you will be tired and want to sleep. You are part of the cycles of the earth and sky, not separate from them. They gently nudge and guide you each day. The sun rises every morning and sets every night. It reaches a peak in the sky just as your meridians reach their peak. All your efforts will be supported if you act according to this cycle. Eat well in the morning, after the sun is up. Sleep well in the dark and let your planning and decision making be wise. Move your body in the light of day, when the pores can open to regulate your heat.

"When one part of the cycle is supported and attended to, it ripples through to all the other parts of the cycle and your system. To eat well in the morning also provides you with freedom during your day. If there are no further opportunities to eat, you have already fuelled your body at the most important time and fed it well. You have also emptied your bowels in the morning so your body can move freely throughout the day. When you are active in the daytime, you will sleep better at night. If you exercise before going to bed your sleep and decision making will be disrupted. If you don't allow yourself some leisure time with those you love and enjoy, what is the purpose of your day? It is a privilege to both work and rest, to toil and play, to be productive and creative, to live and to love.

"When you follow nature's clock, you will function at your best in body, mind, spirit. This is natural. There is no doubt that you will feel better, function better, and be happier. As mentioned before, if there are any impediments or barriers to flow, a practitioner can support you.

"Following the Chinese Clock is accepting your place in the natural world, as part of it. It is acknowledging that your days and your life go through cycles, that the earth and the sky *are* your source of life, that these elements are necessary for your survival.

"You need the sun to provide light and warmth. You need the waters to cleanse, hydrate and to support your flow. You need minerals to sustain your internal functioning; you need food from the earth to nourish you, and you need to grow, shift, and change to avoid stagnation and to create the conditions to thrive.

"Earth, Water, Fire, Metal, and Wood are the sustainers of your life. The earth and sky are your Mother and Father. Every day they are there for you, taking you through the cycles, showing you the way. They will not abandon you. The Chinese Clock is not complicated or rigid. It is as simple as looking outside and knowing where you are."

"Sage, is there additional instruction on the peaks and valleys of meridian times? You have taught us about the function each peak time supports, but how are we to consider the low times?"

"Again, following the clock is easy and simple. The day itself will show you what is needed and support you. It does not take a Sage to instruct you that eating before bed, when you do not need fuel for activities, is unwise; that the night lures you into slumber and not into exercise; that the morning nudges you to new beginnings and anticipation of your day.

"For those of you who enjoy the technicalities, you can look to the times on the clock to mark the peaks and valleys. For those who have lost touch with the natural cycles, this is a good way to begin. Support the meridians during their peak times and they will support you. Respect your meridians during their quiet times and they will work harder than ever for you when their next time in the cycle comes.

"The meridians, you see, are not unlike you. They *are* you!"

Chapter 18

MORE ON FOOD AND THE SEASONS

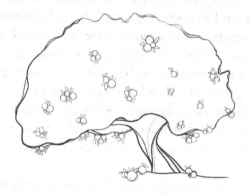

" *age, I am enjoying our time together so much! We have completed the 24-hour cycle of the Chinese Clock but there is so much more I want to learn. I am particularly interested in how we can support nature's patterns of health with respect to food. What foods and food preparations are ideal through the changing seasons? What foods best support our functionality and flow?*"

"Your questions are important. Will you heed the answers? People are always asking about food but they do not follow through with their choices. I hope that what I can offer has a lasting effect upon you, and them.

"Let us consider the sun and the moon. You require the foods of both influences to be well. Food grows and matures according to the changing patterns of the skies, affecting the growth and development of the plants through the seasons. The daytime sun draws food upward and out; the moon helps to build mass and strengthen. When you eat these foods as they are ready, you will grow and develop accordingly. Eating contrary to the season can have consequences in the same way that altered cycles and interrupted flow can breed illness and dysfunction. When energy flows are disturbed or not following nature's cycles, the system is less able to function effectively. This is important.

"Observe the changing phases of growth through the seasons. In the spring the plants are mainly leaves. The roots have not yet developed and are thin and frail. The above-ground green plants are what you need to align with the forces of nature, for nourishment. The colour of spring is green. Eat green foods at this time. In the summer the plants bear fruit—the sweetness of the earth is offered freely. Fruits are mainly composed of water and are what you will need to balance the heat and potential parching of the sun. Eat fruit in abundance when it is abundant. The more time you spend outdoors, under the sun, the more fruit you should eat.

"In the fall and early winter you have root vegetables at their peak of ripeness. It has taken them the full growing season to develop and build their mass. They contain a different type of sweetness than fruit, are more dense, and have less water. They serve to prepare you for winter and carry you through the cold. At this same time the gourds have ripened. They contain a similar sweetness to the root vegetables even though they live above ground. Eat the flesh in the fall and early winter. Dry and save the seeds for the winter months. The nuts and seeds that are abundant in your growing area are easily stored and are one of your protein sources in the intense cold. They are highly dense, compact, and full of life-force energy. Each is the seed of a new plant—an entire crop can be grown from a mere handful. If you want to stay vibrant and strong, ready to burst forth with energy in the spring, you must eat your seeds in the winter. They know how to grow life. It is what they do.

"The herbs of the fields, meadows, and cliffs are seasonal too. Use them when they are in their prime. Spices which are seeds will nourish and strengthen in the winter. They also stimulate and will help you stay warm. You do not need that kind of dense, concentrated energy in the warmer months."

"May I ask about animal protein and its season?"

"Firstly, you should never eat a child animal. To take the life of a child for food is too much to ask of nature.

Just as the plants reach their peak in their own time and season, so do the creatures. It should also be clear, with this one simple teaching, that an old animal of declining strength and life-force will not serve you well either. An animal whose life is taken to support your nourishment and your life should have reached full stature. It should have been living outdoors in the light of the sun and the moon and have eaten the plants in their season. Such animals can offer themselves as a highly concentrated form of nourishment, best eaten during the winter months and colder weather when you need the strength.

"Humans love to play and create. That's what makes them special. All the other creatures are limited to the creation of their own kind—procreation. You contribute your own patterns to those of nature. You create beauty and add complexity. You have the ability to enhance the natural world. You can take the raw materials and use them as a painter uses a canvas. In the case of food, you can create a stew by simmering the bones and meat, adding seasonings, herbs, and root vegetables. What a piece of art a well-crafted stew is! The broth, the flavours, the colours! Don't overdo it. You are using nature's palette to inspire you. Feel what it is you need. Feel what will both serve and delight. Enjoy the craft of food preparation but never let it be a task. Food is a gift of the earth and sky. Food, water, and air are the contributing forces to longevity and your Chi. What greater gift could you receive than the gift that allows your life to continue? It must be received as a gift for the cycles to continue to flow creatively.

"Ah my little apprentice there is much to teach! There is so much beauty in the nourishing gifts of nature. You must take these nuggets of wisdom and start observing for yourself. You must take in the flow and let it sit inside you so you too can know the cycles of nourishment. Do you see? The details are endless and in many ways unimportant. You must now build and grow a knowledge base from this foundation. It is the only way. I will continue to guide but you must be the one who learns."

"Sage, I want to thank you for all your wise teachings. Do you have any parting words for me as I step back and take into my life all that you have offered?"

"Find the art in each moment. Then you will be an artist every day.

"Feel the love in each moment and your world will be filled with love.

"Sense the invisible in each moment and you will balance your physical and spiritual nature.

"Judgements create suffering, for yourself and others. Release judgements and you will experience the bliss of living."

Afterword

I was first introduced to the Chinese Clock in 1999 when I embarked upon a practitioner training program that included Classical Chinese Medicine—Five Element Theory. I found the Clock interesting, fascinating even, but was not drawn to bring it into practice in my daily life. It remained a law that existed as words on a page, showing none of the allure worthy of a dynamic ancient wisdom that could directly influence my ability to be healthy, vibrant, and happy. That came much later.

What did captivate my attention, however, was the beauty, intricacy and complexity of the Five Element approach to healing. Having been a clinical herbalist for more than a decade, it seemed the answer to my dreams. I was an idealist and believed that most people could get well and stay well. I did what I could with herbal medicines, diet, and lifestyle changes, but recognized that I was responding to symptoms when I really wanted to find the root cause. To learn that the ancient Chinese had developed a system of medicine that restored functionality to the human body without pills, herbs, or drugs—that was a revelation!

Classical Chinese Medicine is one of our oldest systems of medicine. It has been documented for more than 2,000 years but is considered at least a thousand years older. Originally called the Five Element Theory of Correspondences, it developed from the premise that a long and healthy life could be achieved by determining what the body needed to function well. At its foundation was the understanding that life is both energy and movement, and furthermore, that life force energy held within it an intelligence of function. We don't teach our bodies how to work: a healthy body does that all by itself. The sages resolved that if the Chi was able to flow fully and held a quality that served, we would be functional in all the ways possible. This was not merely theoretical; it was practical. Through treatment that restores the full flow of Chi, a stomach can return to function, digesting efficiently and effectively. A bowel that appears to have lost its ability to know how and when to eliminate can be nudged back to working normally. Our health and wellness is directly related to our ability to function: to be able to discern what is good for us and what isn't; to not only digest food but to digest our experiences and allow our lives to nourish us; to be inspired by the dawn of a new day; and to connect with others in a loving and kind manner. These and all other aspects of function can be restored.

When I was first introduced to the Chinese Clock it was presented as a chart, showing the names of the meridians and their corresponding times of day. As a practitioner I used it to identify patterns that were arising in patients: what meridian might be linked to waking at the same time each night, or pain heightening at a certain time each day. As the years passed I began to conceive of the Clock in a different way—one that would enable patients to support their own Chi flow between treatments. I discovered that paying attention to one part of the cycle supported the body's ability to heal in other ways. I began to see the Clock as a guide to our own natural "Rhythms of Wellness." Noting that the stomach meridian was at its lowest time in the cycle between 7:00pm and 9:00pm, I asked patients to refrain from eating during this time. Not only did they sleep better and progress faster in their wellness, sometimes old nagging symptoms would disappear. That led me to think, "What if we followed the Clock throughout the day?" Using myself as a test subject, I found that a long-standing symptom of getting up in the night, which had been constant since a kidney surgery 20 years before, resolved within a few months. I never imagined that would happen! When I took a few minutes in the morning to open my meridians before breakfast, I began to feel more lively during the day. Not just in physical energy—I was also happier. This led to a desire to explore the Chinese Clock in greater detail, but the writings I found were limited and based on symptoms that were assigned to individual meridians and not to improvement over the entire cycle.

I believe that what I had stumbled upon was the intended understanding of the power and effectiveness of the Chinese Clock, but that over time, this nuance of its teaching was lost, or at least overlooked. Once this realization sunk in, I began sharing it in earnest. Presented in this way, it made sense to my patients and they actually looked forward to their homework. Hearing their feedback and noting their improvements, I concluded that following the Chinese Clock *is a form of medicine in itself.* To improve our health and functionality we can choose to "synchronize our watches" and be supported by nature to get well. It is an easy system to learn, available to all, free of charge, and is powerful medicine.

I remain intrigued by the thoroughness of the ancient Chinese, their astute brilliance in observation, and the rich cultural tapestry that surely created an ideal environment for this type of knowledge and understanding. In taking you back to the time of the Sages, when the student was privileged to learn directly from the Master, my hope is that it stirred something within you, something ancient and natural, and you too will want to follow the Clock and be well, in all the ways possible.

Appendix: How Do I Begin?

Aligning your daily patterns to the Rhythms of Wellness is a safe, simple, and important way to enhance your physical health as well as your mental/emotional well being. Where and how to begin may be different for everyone, but what follows are some simple guidelines that will also serve as a summary of what has been provided in the preceding chapters. Keep in mind that as the daylight hours change throughout the year, you can adjust accordingly.

Food

The old adage, "Eat breakfast like a king, lunch like a prince, and dinner like a pauper" is consistent with the Chinese Clock. The 'rotting and ripening' meridian, featuring our stomach organ, is at its peak between 7:00 and 9:00am and at its low phase between 7:00 and 9:00pm. Therefore, your digestive capacity will be strongest in the morning and weakest in the evening. It is also advisable to be finished eating (and the initial stages of digesting), 15–20 minutes before the least active phase begins at 7:00pm.

REST AND SLEEP

The functions of 'planning' and those of 'decision making and judgement' begin at 11:00pm and end at 3:00am. Try to be soundly asleep before this phase begins. Also recognize that in areas where the winter is long and dark, you are invited to rest more and sleep longer. Your body will naturally adjust if you allow it.

ACTIVITY

Vigorous activity in the early morning hours before the sun has risen is not recommended. Is it possible to wait until the sun is up and the pores are open so that sweating and the elimination of toxins via the skin can be most productive? In the evening the Fire Element focuses on a different theme, the warmth of connection as opposed to the warmth of heat. Arrange to spend this time of the day with your loved ones, in ways that are enjoyable.

MEDITATION

Many traditions and cultures embodying meditation practices suggest that the early morning pre-dawn hours are optimal, and some specifically state between 3:00 and 5:00am. Knowing that this is the time we are primed to 'receive chi from the heavens' means we can be supported in our meditation practice by following the cycle. Gentle stretching and yoga also opens up the body and the meridian pathways to prepare them for the activity of the day.

KEY FEATURES OF THE DAY:

EARLY MORNING—ideal for meditation and gentle stretching

SUNRISE—watch the sunrise and allow the changing light to activate and align your meridians

MORNING—a hearty breakfast in accordance with your activity levels and needs

MID-DAY—take advantage of the sunlight and spend time outdoors (unless heat is extreme).

EARLY EVENING—eat a light meal and then fast from food until breakfast the next morning

EVENING—spend time with loved ones, focus on activities of the heart, invite joy and laughter

BEDTIME—when preparing for bed allow some time for your eyes to naturally adjust to the changing light as it gets dark outside. Be asleep by 11pm at the latest.

Downloadable Poster: www.jakidaniels.com/books

About the Author

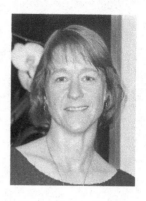

Jaki Daniels lives in Calgary, Alberta, near the foothills of the Rocky Mountains, with her husband Chris. She offers her services through her healing practice, practitioner training program, workshops, and ceremonies, which draw from a life-long passion for healing, and a deep relationship with the natural world and the medicines it holds. She is recognized as a Spiritual Elder in her community, and combines her own experiences with Nature and Spirit with more than 20 years of training with a traditional Cree Elder. Her first two books, *Heeding the Call* and *The Medicine Path*, tell the story of her incredible venture into the medicine-woman style healing ways.

www.jakidaniels.com

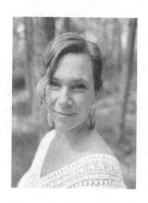

Nancy Kay is a professional artist who creates with oils, acrylic, watercolour and digital art.

As an intuitive channel, Nancy connects with the higher guidance of spirit guides and the angels to bring forth soul messages and imagery.

She is the founder of Juno's Garden and has worked with clients around the world, alchemizing the energy of these visions from spirit into colour, line, and form through her beautiful, one-of-a kind soul art paintings.

To learn more about personalized soul art sessions, and to view Nancy's available art pieces, visit her website.

www.junos.garden